Your Free Gift

I wanted to show my appreciation for your purchase so I have put together a free gift for you!

Easy to follow Get Pregnant Faster Exercise Summary

Just visit

http://newwheelpublishing.com/getpregnantfaster

to download it now

I know you'll love this Gift.

Thanks!

Cecilia Suares

Contents

Introduction

Infertility is not a deficiency. It is a consequence, and like every consequence, it too has a cause. All it takes is for you and your partner to look for it objectively and identify that cause. What you will find is that your lifestyles have drifted far from nature and that has upset the balance that is needed to conceive and bring life to this world.

There are five areas in particular that you need to look at: your source of nutrition; your lifestyle, the balance of your overall body, the relationship you and your spouse have, and most off all, the peace you foster in the home.

These five areas combine to determine if you will have a healthy pregnancy. In traditional and holistic practices, it is believed that the body is very adept at knowing the healthy circumstances of parents before transitioning into fertility. Just like how we are not born fertile, but we grow into it when the time is more opportune to raise a family. The same happens when the age arrives, but if we are not psychologically or physically not prepared for it, the body will control fertility.

To overcome infertility, it requires that you undertake a holistic makeover that includes revitalizing your physical body and rejuvenating your psychology. Remember that infertility is not just a woman's issue, or a man's. It is the two individuals plus the union that they share. An otherwise healthy man and a healthy woman who are not in physical, mental, and emotional union would not always be able to conceive.

This book is designed to walk you through the different phases that will put you and your partner in fertile territory by addressing the five areas identified earlier. What you will also find is that it increases the closeness between you and your partner. This book is really something both of you should read. It creates a responsibility form the beginning that both of you are in this together.

This book is about to change your lives and you will be better off for it. Most people who learn this come back and tell me that, in their hearts, they always knew this to be true but they were blinded by the glitz of commerce and the lifestyle that they were told to lead. But nature always told them otherwise inside. Its just that nature has a very soft and gentle voice that is often drowned out by the chaos of modern civilization.

When I faced infertility we, my husband and I, somehow instinctively knew we needed to return to nature and we allowed that to happen. It changed our lives, blessed us with beautiful, healthy child and brought us together. Infertility was the wakeup call we needed to steer our life back to true happiness. We hope our experience will be of guidance to you as well.

Chapter 1: Toxin Removal Diet

Your first step to fertility involves rethinking your food. You need to remove all the sources of toxins in your body and you need to do that in a gentle way so as to not cause an abrupt destabilization. Take your change in diet slowly and understand that it takes a lot of discipline to do so.

Remove Poultry

Remove all sources of chicken and eggs. Replace your poultry with hardy vegetables and make sure you include tofu and tempeh in your diet. The reduction in poultry intake removes toxins that are found in commercially raised chicken and eggs. The toxins that are in chickens are stored in their flesh and fat, and we ingest them, those drugs are transferred to us. In small quantities, our body is able to handle them, but as the quantities increase, we begin to store them in our fat cells and it begins to take its toll on our overall health. One of the main things that is a problem is the psychological stress that is placed on us without our knowledge.

Remove Beef

The next thing to do is cut out all sources of beef. Beef may not have the toxins found in poultry, but they do have proteins that are not entirely healthy for the body. Beef is also not a natural fit for humans. The problem with beef is that it partially putrefies in the digestive track and creates an unhealthy microbial balance in the gut. The human digestive track is rather long, unlike natural carnivores in the wild that have shorter digestive tracks. Beef also has a high cholesterol content.

When you get rid of beef from the diet, replace it with more fruits especially ones that are usually red when ripe. The aim is to increase your vitamin C intake to help increase the iron absorption that you ingest from vegetables. Vitamin C should go hand in hand with your source of iron because it increases the bioavailability.

Remove Seafood

The next step is to remove fish and seafood from your diet. Replace it with sea weed and other seeds, nuts, and legumes, if you are not already doing it. If you are, just make sure you increase the intake.

Remove Dairy

Finally substitute your dairy, predominantly milk, with nut milk. A good substitute for cow's milk is almond milk or cashew milk.

Recipe Tip: Take half a cup of nuts, wither cashews, almonds, or peanuts, and soak them overnight. Place them in a blender submerged in water and run the blender for 3-5 minutes. Once the nuts are liquefied, strain them in a clean cheesecloth and boil. Add maple syrup and enjoy.

Use Organic Vegetables

Once you have completely replaced all the toxin sources in your diet, make the effort to use organic vegetables and especially ones that are not GMO. This effectively makes you Vegan, but what's in a label? The point is that you are trying to get back to nature and do as your body was designed to do.

Remove Salt

The next thing you need to do is remove salt from the diet. Salt is a toxin that is very dangerous in high quantities. Most people mistake table salt for the salt that the body needs. It is not the same thing. Most of the salt we need, we can get from plant and other food sources. Our electrolytes are not dependent on the salt we use in our cooking. To help remove the salt from your diet, you will have to begin with a liquid fast that lasts 36 hours.

Liquid 36-hour Fast

To do this fast, you need to start three days in advance of the actual day of the fast. Increase your intake of fruits and reduce your grain and carbohydrate intake. By the time you are at the day before the planed fast drink plenty of fluids. On the day before the fast, have your dinner at 7pm and end all solid food from that point.

Once you begin the fast, drink only fruit juices for the next 36 hours and water as well. The fruit juices should be freshly squeezed at home and not purchased from the store. Press the juice just prior to consuming. Do not press batches of it, then leave it in the fridge.

Recipe Tip: Take one banana, an apple, a handful of grapes, and a ripe mango, skin and pit them. Place them in a blender and add ice. Blend until smooth. Strain them in cheesecloth and enjoy. Do not add any sweeteners or salt. You can do this with other combination of fruits as well. Combine citrus fruits, with creamy fruits and crunchy fruits. You can also do the same with vegetables.

Breaking Fast

The next meal you consume will be the morning after the following day. If you keep it up, the breakfast of the morning that you break fast can be done with whole, ripe fruits. Do not consume anything heavy. If for any reason you are not able to get to the 36th hour, if you feel you are about to fall ill, or you get light headed, break the fast with warm ginger tea with a lemon and then start with fruits.

By lunch time you will be ready to eat solid food again. Do this at least once every two weeks. Or if possible, if you are able to do it weekly, you can reduce the fast to 24 hours instead of 36. Once you get past four weeks, reduce the intake to only cool water and not even juices. Keep these fasts to 24 hours and not 36.

24-hour Water Fast

After doing your first 24-hour water fast, you will be ready to remove salt from your diet. The dieting that you have done this far would have strengthened your ideals towards food and begun the removal of toxins from your system. You wouldn't be loosing too much weight, but you would be seeing some loosening of the belt. This is not a bad thing.

The biggest thing you will be able to do here is remove salt from your diet which is a huge step towards balancing your body. Because the next thing that will follow is the reduction of processed sugar.

This is the start of your journey.

Chapter 2: The Mental Picture

Once you have your first phase diet sorted out and you are getting comfortable with it, you need to begin the process of cleansing your mind. We do this with mindfulness achieved through breathing exercises.

Stage 1 Breathing Exercise

The first stage exercise is meant to initiate you into sequence of breathing and mindfulness exercises. There are four stages that you will go through before you begin to see the effects that will astonish you.

The beginning of Stage 1 is simple. Find a spot that you are comfortable with. Close your eyes. You have no other tasks to accomplish. All you have to do is watch your body breathe. When you do this with your eyes closed, it will seem as though you are watching from a point that is between your two eyes, just above the bridge of your nose in the middle of your forehead. It will only seem like this. Identify this as the seat of your Self.

Once you close your eyes and start watching your breathing, remember that that's all you need to do. Remember to place all other distractions on hold. When you sit down and watch your breathing, count how long it takes to inhale. 1 Mississippi ... 2 Mississippi... 3 Mississippi... until your breath reaches the end of its natural cycle, and prepares to exhale. Remember, you are only watching, not controlling. So whatever rhythm of breathing that is currently a part of you, is what you are watching. Do not try to change it to inhale deeply or exhale fully.

When you do this you will note the number of seconds it takes to inhale. Then count the time it takes to exhale. The time it takes to exhale, may or may not be the same time as the inhale, and for now that does not matter. What you need to do is just be aware of the count. Keep doing this and focus on the breath and the count.

When you are done, open your eyes and relax in your same position and slowly let the rest of life enter your conscious observation. Listen to each sound as they enter your consciousness. Then open your eyes and let the information flood you.

As you become aware of your surrounding, keep in mind only what you must. Because you have just begun to realize that when you are flooded with information, your mind can only pay partial attention to any one thing. Let this be a lesson on the path to healing and getting ready for becoming a parent.

When you repeat this everyday for a week, you will do two things: you will slow down your rhythm and you will peel away whatever stress you are currently facing, even if you didn't know you had any. But this is just the first part of it. To understand nature, slowing down is a major part of success.

Stage 2 Controlled Breathing

The second part is when you begin to control your breathing to match the inhale and exhale times. By matching the times you are intentionally controlling your breathing. But do not jump to this step right away. You must take it slow. The chances are, that you are like the 99% of people around the world and your breathing techniques are wrong to begin with. If you learnt to breath right from young, your diaphragm will be strong and you can control your tempo incredibly well.
As you practice this breathing technique what you will slowly realize aside from the better breathing habits and the calming of you mind, you will also notice that your extremities begin to tingle. It just means that your pulse oxygen level is going up. You are sending more oxygen to the rest of your body and they are literally waking up.

With this simple exercise, and without too much effort, you have already begun to cleanse your body and oxidize much of the gaseous toxins that are present. By doing the weekly water fast, you have also started to cleanse your gut, and by doing that, you have started to improve the quality of your blood. With the increased blood quality and the increase breathing, oxygen is going to be flowing in abundance, and your cells will begin to rejuvenate themselves. The increased Vitamin C from the fruits you are now taking in replacement of the meat, is also helping your immune system to boost its performance.

Point to Note: The effort to get pregnant is by no means just the responsibility of the woman, or just the man. It is up to both of you to conceive, protect the pregnancy, and bring the child into this world and care for it. It is also important then that you do this exercises together. After all it is for the betterment of your future family.

Kick the Smoking Habit

At this point in time, if either of you are smoking, it is time to kick the habit. You cannot hope to get pregnant if one of the things that one or both of you are doing is pumping nicotine and tar into your body.

Stage 3 Visualize Your Distractions

If you have managed to quite smoking, the third stage of meditation is going to be able to help you completely quit the habit and get you on the road to health. The third stage is also rather simple and all you need to do is extent the time you take away for the purpose of meditation.
The idea here is to visualize your distractions, and smoking is certainly a distraction. When you get to this stage what you are doing is to acknowledge your distractions, but not taking part in them. You will find that your thoughts have a mind of their own. Those thoughts are beyond your self and what you are doing is

separating your self from random fragments of thought. Don't worry - everybody has them.

When you are watching your breathing you will realize that you are able to monitor everything that goes on about you. The same thing is now expanded when you start to look at not just what you are doing with your breath but also what you are doing within your mind. The thoughts that you have will be more visible to your minds eye and you will be able to watch them go by without interacting with them.

The benefit of this third stage is that you are becoming the master of your mind which means that you will be able to be less stressed in many situations. To really reap the benefits, you should keep going and never stop the daily meditation routine and the weekly fasting.

Just as fasting and veganism cleanses the body, mindfulness, and breathing exercises cleans the mind.

The mindfulness exercises that you have been practicing allow you to remember one salient truth that the past and the future do not matter and what does matter is the moment. Being mindful is about being in the moment. Being in the moment is the most important thing in the world when you are trying to do anything in this world.

When you and your spouse are in the midst of making love, as you are trying to conceive after a difficult time, do not think about all the times that it didn't work out. Do not think about that time that you think you are ovulating. Don't chase the clock or the base temperature to feel if you are at the right second. Do not force your husband to get it right, down to the last micro second. That is not the way one gets pregnant. When you want to get pregnant there is only one thing that matters and that is your spouse. You turn 100% of your mind's energy, your mindfulness onto your spouse and both of you need to be in the moment and not on what ifs.

Stage 4 Instantaneous Focus

When you get to this stage the idea is to be able to control your breathing at the drop of a dime - to control what your mind is doing at the drop of a dime - to control where you are in a moment. And once you can do all that, you have reached the pinnacle of the simple meditation. There is no need to visualize anything. Your breath is the most powerful thing in the world. Between your mind, and your breadth, there is almost nothing that you cannot cure. In stage four, it is time to move your meditation to other parts of your life. Where ever you are, pay full attention to what you are doing. This practice comes in handy when the day comes that you finally conceive and now your kid is a toddler, you will find that your mindfulness on your new angel, will create a bond between the two off you that can never be severed.

Where ever you are, make sure you are in the moment. Whether you are on the bus, on a plane, be mindful. Being mindful is not about being withdrawn. You are fully aware of all that is happening around you. You are just not participating, but you are watching.

Point to Note: When I was pregnant and kept up my meditation, during the second trimester I focused in on a thought of my yet unborn child. We had already formed a strong bond. My meditation times would usually include my baby, and during one of these sessions, I had an image flash before my mind's eye and as I followed it, I got a good look at the baby in my arms. I remembered the face and when my child was born, she had the exact same face that I had seen in my thoughts. It was better than any ultrasound I had ever known.

Meditation has a multi dimensional effect on mothers and fathers. It is one of the best ways to get in touch with what is going on inside you. With mindfulness exercises and breathing exercises one of the benefits you will begin to experience is that your body will tell you what it needs. This will result in you getting visions of what is necessary and what you need to eat. It will be the way your body tells you what it needs from a nutritional standpoint. It may even tell you what you will need to get pregnant.

Those are the possible side effects, but what you are shooting for is mostly to get rid of the mental toxins that plague you. It will reduce the stress and it will also be a way for you to learn not to take on more stress. By the time you are done you will be able to be calm and collected. It will even help you during natural child birth.

Chapter 3: Physical Work Out

If you're not regularly working out, you should get started now. The best time to get your workout regimen going is around the time you start thinking of starting a family. Your workout routine must be vigorous, to increase your metabolism and your breathing, while being able to work a balanced set of muscle groups.

Running

Running is the most natural and the most beneficial for anyone and if you are a morning person, a good run to start the day will increase your stamina and your metabolism for the entire day.

Keep your run constant at 30 minutes where the first 7 minutes is to warm up. The following 12 minutes is for high-burn runs, where you run fast and you focus on your breathing. The next 4 minutes is for a slower pace where you get to catch your breath and then you do a sprint for about a minute. Finally, the last six minutes is for you to cool down, reduce the pace and let your body catch up. Do this for about a week and you will notice that your entire day changes. You will be able to breath better and you will be able to enjoy your meals better too. What's more, you will be able to sleep more soundly as well.

Dress warm if it's in the winter and dress light if it is in the summer. The idea is to keep your body at the optimal metabolic level. Make sure you hydrate well and keep your muscles warm. Once you get past the first ten days of doing this daily, you will be able to increase the pace across the entire segment. For instance, if you covered 1 mile in the first 7 minutes, this week its time to increase the distance to about 1.2 miles. You can use Google map to plot your run. Just get the area where you live on the map, mark out the distances and you will know where you need to be running at a particular speed.

Once you've increased it in the second week by 20% across the board, take some time to get used to the increased pace. Then increase it by another 20% the following week until you are not able to increase it anymore. Once you get to this point, keep it steady and run your course everyday. There is no need to increase it any longer.

Running should be the core of your workout. When you run, try not to listen to music. It is apart of the mindfulness exercise. Listening to music while you run may make the run more manageable, but the intent of the run is more than just to get physically fit, it is also meant to keep you mentally fit too. By being mindful of the run, you accomplish two things at once: the workout; and the practice of being mindful. You must learn to be present at each step, at each point your heel meats the road, at each breath that refreshes your lungs and at each step you make your way home.

Perspiration

Another important reason you want to work out is that perspiration is a tremendous opportunity to remove toxins that have been stored. Whenever you ingest toxins, it gets into your blood stream, then transferred to the fat that is created that day and stored in your tissue. It will stay there for a long period of time, until the fat cells are called into service. The moment they are called to ranks, and the fat is converted to energy, the toxin that was stored there is released into the blood stream.

When you get pregnant, you will begin the process of losing weight for one reason or another. The toxins that you have accumulated, will be released and it will have an effect on the fetus. If you have ever smoked pot for any period of time or done harsh contraband, then you need to do a lot of workouts to expel any toxins that are still stored in your fat cells.

If you decide that running is hard on your knees, a good

replacement would be to cycle. Cycling imparts the same level of activity for your heart and muscle groups as running and you will have the same benefits. To make thing fun, you could cycle and run in alternating sequence.

Chapter 4: Massage

Just as workouts aid the body in increasing blood flow and endorphin release, massages are also an effective way to get the blood flowing into areas that are either 'blocked' or not receiving enough oxygen supply. Massages tend to squeeze out endorphins from muscle groups that are not fully functioning.
For instance when you predominantly run for the your work out, it is very likely that you back, shoulder and forearm muscles are under developed compared to your legs and lower body. When this happens you will build up a store of endorphins and lesser blood flow to the upper body. This is usually fine, but to optimize your health it's advisable to have massages to tenderize the stiff muscles and release those endorphins. It also unblocks and revitalizes your upper frame.

In the same way, if you are constantly doing push ups and pumping iron, but not running, then you are going to be in a situation where the upper body is going to be releasing all your endorphins, but you are not going to be releasing anything from your lower body. For this instance then you should do massages to the part of your body that you are not working out.
There are numerous massages that you can do and many of them will help purge toxins stored in the fat cells and in the musculature. A deep tissue massage is a good way to help remove toxins from the body and relive it of blockages that reduce proper blood flow, nutrition delivery, and oxygen availability. It also helps to reduce the gas, like nitrogen and carbon dioxide, in the parts of your body that are not constantly moving.

Deep Tissue Massage

The massage you should have after you have done at least one month's worth of weekly 24-hour water fasts and at least one week's worth of exercise, is the deep tissue massage. The deep tissue massage is not going to be entirely blissful at first, but you will only feel the benefit at the end of the second or third session. Ideally, you should have your partner give you this massage, but do not end this massage sexually.

Feet

The massage starts at the feet. Lie flat, face forward and remain relaxed. Have your partner begin by squeezing your toes gently as though he is ringing our a sponge. He is in fact doing just that. He is squeezing the tissue that make up your feet and releasing whatever is stored there including gas, liquid and toxins. He is pushing the endorphins out of this area as well so that new hormones can replace it. He should press them to the point where it starts to hurt a little. You could communicate to him when it hurts.

This is also a good practice for the two of you to bond at a level that is not common between today's modern couple. A massage is a highly intimate bonding of two people and this, whenever possible, should not be done by a stranger.

The toes should be stretched to the limit of their travel and they should be moved from one limit to the other gently but with strength. This does two things, it allows you the benefit of loosening your tissue, and it teaches him the limit of strength to use on you.

Once the toes are done, it is time to focus on the arch of the foot. This is an important part of the leg as there are a number of nerve endings here that can stimulate the rest of the body. The nerve endings need to be stimulated by the use of the knuckles and the middle phalange of the index finger.

Use the knuckle of the index finger to gently rub the arch from the direction of the toe to the heel. Do this to the point of moving from the big toe to the little toe. Spend at least five minutes here on each leg. Once this is done, us the thumbs of the two hands and push the flesh of the arch outwards. The left thumb moving up and to the left and the right thumb moving up and to the right.

From the feet, push the blood up the calf then press down on the ball of the calf with both palms side by side, longitudinally. Press this until you feel a sensation of pleasure. This is the release of the endorphins stored in the calves.

Then articulate the lower leg at the knee and push it all the way back, as far as possible, until the knee is able to stretch. Attempt to bend it till the heel touches your gluteus maximus. This will also have positive sensations as the endorphins are also released form the thigh muscles as they are stretched.

Thighs

Massage the fleshy area just above the knees. There are lymph nodes located here and massaging them will release the lymphatic fluids and clear out any blockages. Find the location with the thumb and gently, in circular motion, massage the lymph node at the knee area. This may be a little uncomfortable as you might also be pressing the lower femoral nerve. Be careful not to press the nerve too much. If there is an inordinate amount of discomfort, do tell you partner.

Take a 2-minute break and have some warm water to drink and resume the massage. Continue the upward track until you reach the hip's iliac crest.

While your partner is massaging your lower limbs, and while he continues up toward the rest of your body, you should focus on the present. Do not let your thoughts wander or leave the room you are in. Be mindful of the present, always using your breath to anchor the consciousness to your center of gravity.

Many proponents of massages also advice using soothing music to increase the effect. In actuality, you do not need the music.

Music, candles, and perfume are distraction that allow you and your partner to escape the moment to a moment that is not real. The perfume of the candles, the aroma of the scented sticks and oils are all escapes of the present. You are trying to be in the moment, not the other way around. So make sure there is no music and no scented candles. Make sure there is no perfume other than the natural smell of the oils that you are using and the natural smell of each other.

Question: Do you know what the natural scent of your partner is? Does he know yours?

Your partner's natural smell is not that of some designer fragrance. You need to get past that. When your child is born, make sure you do not use and fragrances. Your natural skin smell is one that he will look for and will be able to recognize, do not deprive him or her of that.

Many people who do this program, begin by feeling self conscious of their body odor. If you have been following the regimen thus far, by turning vegan, fasting, and working out, your body would, by now, have reached a stage where your natural odor is prominent and it will be on the sweeter side than on the pungent.

The problem with today's population is that our body odor is a reflection of what we eat and when we eat toxic food, our perspiration carries these putrefying toxins and it lands up in unpleasant body odor, which we then try to cover up with deodorants and perfumes. Once you resort to your natural self, you will even find that the odors that made you self-conscious after a work out are no longer there.

Returning to the Massage

While you receive the massage, remain in the moment and continue to breath. Feel your body, absorb the person with you, his smell, his touch, his presence. Feel the warmth of his hands and feel the texture of his touch. This is what you need to bond with the father of your children.

Pelvic Area

The pelvic area is rich in lymph nodes and deserves to be massaged gently, but applying a firm amount of pressure. Do not press to hard, but at the same time do not remain only on the surface. Massage from the center, outwards.

Back

With the hips complete, leave the vaginal area. It does not need to be massaged. Then move on to the back. Press down on the back, applying pressure, then releasing, Each cycle of application and release should be done with progressively more force, yet gracefully. The force would come to point of pleasure, then mild discomfort, then become heavy. Notify your partner where the pressure is and when it starts to become uncomfortable. Each time the pressure is applied and released. You will feel a surge of pleasure coursing through your body.
The back is the unsung hero of the woman's body. We tend to carry a lot of our baggage here. We do not have the upper body strength of the males in our species so everything falls to the center of our frame. It is also the place that supports our pregnancy. Those with soft backs or inadequate back support will find it extremely difficult to conceive as the body knows it is not in good shape to manage an extra 25 pounds (including the fluids) in the belly that will soon expand. Even healthy women have a problem with this.

Rub the downward and outward after the pressure application. Use both hands, starting at the spine and using the palm to push outwards.

Rear Shoulders

When you arrive at the shoulders use the squeezing motion that was done on the calves and the legs. Pressing the areas of the lymph nodes in the front of the shoulders. This also leads to the neck. Most of you who have any form of iron deficiency will usually complain of back and neck aches after a long day. Massaging the shoulders here may seem adequate, but what you really should do is press the shoulders only after massaging the lower limbs. The increase of endorphins in the blood, will increase the oxygen to the area of your back and neck and you will instantly be relieved of that crick in your neck.

This is the end of the massage for the deep tissues. You will end this massage with a drink of pure, room temperature water. Hot water or cold water are not preferable as it changes the ambient temperature of your core.

When you do this correctly, you will notice that there is a change in the color of your urine. What used to be stained before your vegan and fasting days will, after the deep tissue massage, be slightly greenish. Do not be alarmed, you are just pushing the toxins once stored in your muscles. After four sessions this phenomena will stop and your release will return to being clear again.

If it is your time of the month, you can still do the massage if you are comfortable, and if you partner is comfortable. There is nothing to be disconcerted about. This massage is a must to begin with and it will form the basis of all the other massage regimens. The idea of this massage is to clear the lymphatic system and release endorphins. It is also designed to increase blood flow to the limbs, and the lower back as well as the hips.

Chapter 5: Meditation II

The first round of meditation exercises in Chapter 2, gave you an introduction to how to reconnect to your Self. Your Self is the consciousness that resides in the body and is connected to the physical body by the breathing that you do. Whenever you feel a source of tension present, return to your breath and watch how it anchors your Self to the present and the moment. The key to everything is the breath that anchors the mind.

Once you have mastered the techniques listed in Chapter 2, you will find many doors that open up to the inside of you. The proverbial flood gates will open and you will be able to see life differently than you have been all this while.

Reasons for Getting Pregnant

One of the keys to overcoming infertility to for you to understand the reasons why you are desirous of becoming pregnant. Your desires need to be pure and unselfish. If you are forcing yourself to be pregnant because you think that's what is expected of you, or if you have any other ulterior motive, that will show up in your meditation. You need to deal with those issues before you can move further.

Remember, the fact that you are not conceiving says a lot about what is going on inside. There is nothing wrong with you other than the fact that your Self knows that something you are doing in the present and in the recent past, has made it unwise for you to have a child. You need to resolve that and you need to do it during your meditation techniques.

There are two layers here that you need to find and resolve. One is the superficial you that wants to be pregnant almost just to prove that you are a women. Especially for those of you who initially found it hard to get pregnant, the desire to get pregnant has evolved and it is not at a point where you need to prove to the world, your in-laws, your husband, and even to yourself that you are a fully functioning woman.

You are. You just need to overcome the blocks and the hurdles.

The key to this meditation is to increase the strength of your Self. The self is the consciousness that you were introduced to in Chapter 2. It is the consciousness that was watching the breathing and watching all the distractions and whatever was going on while you were watching your breathing. It is different for the thoughts that pop up. It is different from the distractions that catch your attention. It is the one that has control over what actions you take. This is the seat of your personal power. You need to find it and activate it.

Center of Mass

To do this, you need to imagine your center of gravity as a large mass. When you sit down to breath, take a deep breath, a few deep breaths to consolidate all that is happening and you will see this breath anchors to what feels like the center of your chest. You will suddenly feel a mass of stability in the middle of you torso. Focus on this stability and ponder on it. Revel in it, it will make you feel strong. Imagine this weight to be pure energy and whatever form of energy you see in your imagination, let that be the symbol of your center mass.

Many people see a flame when they imagine their center and energy. You can use the flame as your symbol too, except remember that is just symbolical. The real feeling cannot be expressed within the confines of language.

By this point you begin your meditation in a dark room without the distraction of sound, without the distraction of worry, anxiety and thoughts. The first round of breathing exercises have thought you how individually your mind works and what works for you when you get distracted. Apply that every time you move away from your center of mass. The best way most people who do this feel is that they return to breathing and center their energy.

The Flame

If you imagine your energy as a flame, then let your imaginary forces fan the flame to increase it to a point where it envelopes your chest and spreads to your mind's eye - the seat of your Self. Just as the breath anchored your mind to your body, the flame will fuse your body to your Self. Doing this ignites the deepest sense of unity between your Self and your physical body, which up to now was never in harmony. Which is why you did things that would harm your body without taking any note of it.

Something to think about: Why else would someone do something to harm his or her own body, just so the brain could feel pleasure?

The practice of this kind of meditation places you back in harmony with your body. When you are in harmony with your body, you will know what is wrong with your body and you will be your best council. The unification of mind and body is a powerful combination only bested by the unification of two individuals unifying to bring forth a new life. But to get to that point, you need to get past the barrier that exists between your Self and your body.

The constant practice of imagining the energy that flows from the centre of your mass, then developing into energy that can be visualized as a flame will result in something that you can connect with and move from your center to your Self. When you practice this enough, you will fuse the two parts.

This will result in the triumvirate of the body. You will have your Self, your body and your breath all united. From this point of the meditation, aided by the cleansed body, and the alert mind, you will find that you are one step closer to understanding the reason behind your seeming infertility.

It is important that you continue your water fast, it is important that you are still vegan and it is important that you and your partner continue the massages to help the bonding. Ideally, everything that you are doing, your partner should be doing too. It is also ideal that you massage your partner in the same way he massaged you. When you both reach the point of meditation that we've this far described, it would be beneficial that both of you sit in the room together, meditating.

Combined Meditating

Combined meditating is when both of you, who have been thus far exercising separately, and meditating separately begin to come together and begin your meditation together. This is almost a spiritual experience for those who do this frequently. Not only will you feel your own flame when you meditate, you will begin to feel the flame of the person in the room with you. It may even be distracting as you do this for the first few times, but remember the thing that gets you out of distraction is the breathing that anchors you back to your center of mass. The breathing, by this time in the process, has become so graceful that you turn to it instinctively and it will always bring you back to where you want to be.

When you learn how to breath, it will even help you in your childbirth, especially those of you considering natural childbirth. So make sure you always look at your breath.

When you engage in combined meditation, it is a deeply personal experience. You are letting someone into the very depths of your soul and it transcends the physical relationship that prepares you for a new level of sexual experience which will be covered in the next phase.

Most women cry after the first sexual experience and never understand why. Reasons that have been offered up by many is that there is a chemical change or that they feel regret. The real reason is that the sexual experience is supposed to be a unification of two souls. It is the act that brings two beings together to form a third being. It is a deeply spiritual union that has been trivialized by the discipline of marketing. We all pay the price for this.

To get over the effects of it, the combined meditation will step across all boundaries and result in a unification of two people who were once separate beings, and now making it into one. The combined meditation is not like synchronized swimming,

Begin by getting comfortable in the room, turn the lights down. The room should be ventilated with fresh air and it should be a cool environment. It should be comfortable. Dress lightly. The best clothes to dress in are pure cotton that is unbleached. It allows for airing and keeping ventilated.

Do not use incense sticks or aroma oils. Do not have any music playing in the background. You can sit facing each other or back to each other but do not sit too far away or too close. You should sit at the boundary of your individual personal spaces. Do not touch each other because you do not want to distract the spiritual contact you are about to make with the physical contact of touch.

Both of you can begin simultaneously but it is not a necessity, in fact do not make plans of starting that way because that in itself will be a distraction. Once you begin, and your partner begins, you will start of at to different points in time and space. That is fine, but you will meet as the two of you approach the point of meditation.

Begin with the breathing exercises and move on to anchoring your Self to the center of energy. Once you are anchored, transmit the energy to the Self and hold it here. When you get there, if you partner is also at the same stage, you will see that there is an abundance of energy in the room and you will feel the glow and the warmth that only your Self can perceive. If you were to open your eyes, the room will remain in the same level of illumination as you left it when you started.

The level of illumination that you are perceiving in your Self is the combined energy of two individual beings. What you perceive and meet will not be recognizable to you in definable terms but you will know that it is your partner. Remain focused on this energy and you will see it intensify.

Do remember that you may not achieve this state the first time you do this, or the second time. Most of my students who do this, do however, achieve it before getting to the fifth time and it gets deeper with practice.

By this time you will know your partner in more ways that you would have ever imagined. He is the father of your child. She is the mother of your child. The connection that you make from a physical, mental and energetic level will be nothing that can ever be matched by any other relationship in the past, present or the future. The stronger your bond to your spouse, the higher the possibility of pregnancy and the higher the possibility of a sublime child.

Focus on making a child born of love, not out of sex.

The unification of two people that can reach this level is something that will open up your body to the ability to conceive. It is the way that your body makes contact with your spouse and instead of you forcing the pregnancy, your body will crave the pregnancy. That the position you want to be in where your body, and every fiber of your being, is inline with your Self and the only thing that all parts of you want, is to conceive a child with the spouse that you are bonded to.

Chapter 6: Doing it at Home

This chapter is a slight departure from the flow of things as it has occurred thus far. This chapter is a bit of a pause to the reading you have thus far done. Here we will go over some healing practices that you will make in the kitchen and some oils that you can prepare for the use in cooking and for use in massages.

Making Oil at Home

One of the greatest challenges to cooking wholesome food is the oil we use to prepare meals. The unimaginable thing about these oils we find at the grocery store are meant to be put in our food, but aren't even good enough to rub on our skin, because it could cause an allergic reaction or may just be unhealthy. Some of the oils that come packaged are even carcinogenic if inhaled. Imagine that.

So the alternative is to make oil at home and it is not that difficult as you may think. The favorites can be categorized as nut oils or seed oil. Nut oils are my favorite. The process is the same for both. All you need is a nut oil extractor. It usually comes with a hand crank and is made of solid cast iron. You can shop around for that online. Just take something like peanuts, almonds, or cashew nuts and place them in the hopper and start cranking. In no time you will start to see the oil being pressed out into the container. The oil in 100% natural, as you pressed it yourself, and if you bought organic nuts, the oil is as healthy as it gets.

There is another way of preparing oil that does not require any purchase. If you go to the Asian food market, you will find that they sell fresh old coconuts. The coconut must be aged and not young. The flesh of young coconuts will not have the oil you need. When you get the aged coconuts, scrape the hard flesh out and grate it. Take the grated coconut and add hot water to it and squeeze it.

What you will see is a white liquid that will flow. Place that in a clean container and in the refrigerator. By the following day, the water would have separated from the cream and the cream would have solidified because of the cold. Scoop the cream and place it on a warm pan. As the cream renders you will find that it oozes oil. Use a strainer and separate the grain from the oil and store the oil in the fridge.

You can use this oil to lightly sauté vegetables or to garnish your salads. It is highly aromatic. If you are on the heavy side of the bathroom scale, then do not use coconut oil in your food. If you have oily skin, also, do not use it in food. But you can use it for your massages.

Soaks

There is one particular water therapy that I have found effective. It was developed in the late 19th century and is called a Kuhn Bath. This is an amazing discovery and when we found it we made some modifications to it. But the essential idea is still developed from the theories of Louis Kuhn.

The Kuhn bath is simple to do and very effective at relieving a number of ailments. In fact if you have a constipation problem, this is one way that you could relive it naturally. It also works well if you are having problems conceiving.

In your tub, fold a towel in half five times till you have something thick enough to comfortably sit on, or if you have a rubber donut, that would be ideal. Place that in the tub and fill it with cold water. Do not use warm water for this. Full the tub to about 12 inches above the seat you've prepared and once the water is filled, remove your clothes and sit naked in the tub.

Clay Packs

One of the most effective natural infertility practices you can do to unclog the uterus is to use a mud pack at least three times a week. If you have irregular periods, and that is suspected of being one of the causes of the infertility, then you do not have much to worry about. The clay packs have a way of helping the body to work the uterus to its normal state. The process is very simple. Find earthen clay. Most people will find it in their front yard if they dig down deep enough. It is orange in color and is dense. Get about a pound of clay and wrap it in a swaddle cloth made of cotton and tie it around your naval. Leave the pack there for 30 minutes.

Mud Packs

Do the same things with mud packs to the back. Place clean mud in cotton swaddle cloth and wrap it around your back. This will relieve the nerves in the back that are knotted due to tight muscles. The relief is immediate.

Ginger Tea

Use young, fresh ginger. Slice some from the rhizome and seep it in boiling water for the time it take the boiling water to cool to a temperature that you can sip the tea. The tea is a good way to cleanse the system and it helps with relieving your cravings of salt and sugar.

Home Made Milk

Soak either soy beans, cashews, or almonds in fresh clean water and remove the shell or casings. Blend them in the processor for 3-4 minutes or until the nut has been reduced to a paste. Keep adding water slowly - a few tablespoons at a time. It will become a paste. Once it becomes a smooth paste, you can add water till it turns creamy. Then add one more cup of water from that point and place it in a pan to boil. That additional cup is to account for evaporation during heating. Add sweetener that is appropriate for your body.

You will find that there is nothing that you can't make at home. Everything from oil to even sugar if you need it. Whatever you can't make at home you probably do not need. Cheese is not something that your body needs to keep healthy. So do not worry about making those. Switch to tofu and you will begin to feel better.

Chapter 7: Aroma Therapy

Aroma therapy can get a little controversial these days only because it has become such an industry and everybody seems to be hopping on to the bandwagon. The confusion exists, and is understandable, because aroma therapy attaches its cure to the senses and then creates a desire for something that is pleasant.

Enjoying the aromas of a beautiful spring morning is natural and it is uplifting. Just as enjoying the smell of a late spring rain shower can be invigorating. Your aroma therapy should be limited to everything that is natural and nothing that comes pre-packaged in a bottle. The aroma of nature returns the body to its peaceful center.

Natural Aroma

What do you consider to be natural aroma? Natural aroma is the smell of nature around you. Everything that is not man made and releases an aroma is natural. Even decay of a tree in the forest, when it mixes with the dew of the morning is refreshing. The same can't be said for the exhaust of car. The ocean breeze that has a salty aroma is nature. The smell of a leather tannery upwind is not.

Natural aroma has a direct impact on the body's ability to conceive naturally. Unnatural aroma has the reverse. If you want to lift your senses with the use of chamomile, then buy the flowers and smell those. If you want to smell a potpourri of cinnamon and cloves, then do the herbs yourself and those would work great at lifting your spirits during the course of the day. However, keep your bedroom and your meditation free form aroma.

The reason for this is to get you and your partner to recognize the smell of each other. You will notice that you can recognize them in a room even when you are not looking. That's how strong your senses are when you do that.

Pets

Promote your natural odor in the home especially when the baby is born so that the baby feels constant security. Try not to have pets in the house for the same reason, because their odor will overwhelm yours and there will be a confusion of smells because you would then have to get deodorizers to make the house smell less like your dog. If you have a cat, that is worse because cats can sometimes release bacteria that reduce your chances of getting pregnant. For those of you who want to have cats after having a child, think twice because handling cat feces in a house that has babies is highly dangerous for the infant.

Essentially pets are not the best things in the home, or apartment, but they are great if you have a ranch or a large compound where they can be one with nature as well.

Not having a pet also serves as a psychological purpose. The reason we have pets is because we transfer the inborn desire to nurture offspring to the pet. Once that desire has been satiated, then the real desire to have a human baby is also diminished. Keep the desire pent up in you to have baby, not a pet. There is a huge difference, and keeping a pet in the house is not good for you, or the pet.

Coming Back to Aroma Therapy

Aroma therapy is a misnomer, unless you use natural ingredients. Each aroma that is in its natural state, not burned or boiled has its benefits. Incense, other aroma products are the by-product of burning something and within that smoke would be a smorgasbord of chemicals that will become a part of your breathing. It is no less harmful than breathing in haze from a forest fire. The contents are the same.

In aroma therapy there are some natural scents that are beneficial to the safe feeling that you can get used to. The first is your spouse's natural body aroma. When your spouse travels, keep a shirt that he has worn next to you so that you get a good nights rest as you sleep. When you are pregnant and he is away, do the same and the baby would appreciate it.

Do not use scented candles as they contain numerous toxins. You could use green fauna in the house as they contain natural smells that would provide peace, but flowers are not encouraged as it contains pollen and that may upset the delicate aroma balance of the home.

The same goes for soaps and shampoos. Keep them as perfume free as possible. The chemicals are harsh on your skin to begin with and it douses your natural scent. Instead, use perfume free soaps and shampoos. Do the same for the laundry as well and sun dry them when possible, or use an effective clothes dryer that will remove the moisture effectively from the clothes. The possibility of leaving them wet and attracting mold is not something you want to contend with. Mold and the toxins it releases are detrimental to your effort to overcome infertility naturally.

The idea of rejecting perfumes and artificial deodorizers may seem completely strange. But you will find that your body odor has considerably diminished and most likely abated. Even your bowel movements have little to no odor. Your cooking in the kitchen is also less obnoxious. Perfumes were designed to cover the odor of a healthy body.

Chapter 8: Maintenance Diet

In Chapter 1 we looked the change in diet to rid the body of the toxins that may have built up over the years of neglect and misguided ideals. Now that your body has returned to what it naturally should be, we now need to increase your health so that you can get above the curve. If you were considered to be behind the curve when you were unable to get pregnant, the diet and everything that you did in the last few chapters has allowed you to get on the curve. Now the maintenance diet is going to put you ahead of the curve.

Understanding the Woman's Body

We must accept that just as all women are not the same, neither are our physiologies, our thoughts, our predilections, or our avocations. One way to look at determining an individual's diet is to look at the way food affects them and the way they react to it. This is called the nutritional balance. With the proper nutritional balance, a person's energy will increase and their health and vitality will be at the highest possible. When a person is imbalanced they will feel their worst and that has a psychological impact that is a significant barrier in achieving pregnancy. The nutritional balance of all women can be categorized into three groups: light, heavy, and spirited. This nutritional balance is at the root of almost all we do, and who we are.

LNB

Visualize someone like Catherine Zeta-Jones or Oprah Winfrey. Here are two women who fall under the category of the light nutritional balance (LNB). It is not a function of their mind, but its what they are born with. It manifests itself in certain visual cues such as larger frames, smoother skin, and their characteristics are typified by easy weight gain, sluggishness and lethargy, fluid retention, yeast infections, and lack natural motivation.

HNB

The second category, heavy nutritional balance (HNB), includes those of you who have the body frame of someone like say, Mia Hamm, Jennifer Aniston, or Sharon Stone. This profile typically results in a personality that is prone to hot tempers and irritability, hot flashes, and night sweats, as well as heavy menstrual flows.

SNB

That leaves the rest of us who are similar in body frame to Nicole Kidman, Cameron Diaz or Halle Berry. If you are share a similar body frame and are prone to nervousness, anxiety, panic, mood swings, vaginal dryness, constipation, bloating, and joint aches, then you are spirited nutritional balance (SNB).

How we fine tune our diets based on our nutritional balance is what will catapult our ability to reach a higher level of peace and eventually achieve fertility. With that as our launching pad, we can then analyze diet, lifestyle, and rest. The first thing now is for you to determine your metabolic profile.

Fine Tuning the Diets

There are three diets that will individually be able to bring balance to the forces within you. Because each of us has a different constitution and the chemistry that results is not entirely uniform, we find that the best way to prescribe the balancing diets is to look at the fruits, vegetables, legumes, seeds, nuts, oils, and spices.

The LNB Diet

LNBs are best balanced by eating foods that stimulate the mind and soul. LNBs are best suited to foods that are astringent, bitter and spicy. The spiciness helps clear the mental fog while the bitter will help to keep the blood sugar stable and the astringent will reduce the propensity to retain water.

You are already refraining from sweeteners, but if you have yet to kick the habit, you should realize that you are highly susceptible to insulin spikes and you need to put a stop to that. If you are having trouble letting go of sugar, remember that sugar and salt play together. If you have sugar, you will crave salt and vice versa. To kick the habit sip ginger tea all day. The recipe is in Chapter 6.

The reason LNBs love their sugar is because their natural sluggish self have always felt energized when they have some sugar and they are attracted to the burst of energy, but that just makes the cycle more viscous. Use honey to increase your energy levels, if you need to. But the exercise in the earlier chapters will get you up and about more then the sugar can. In addition to the honey, you are more than welcome to supplement your sugar intake with natural sweet fruits that have a low glycemic index. The following are great ways to introduce the healthy sugars that you need: berries, cherries , apricots, grapes purple, raisins, guava, pears, cranberries, apples, prunes, pomegranates, dry figs, and peaches.

Vegetables

To keep yourself in balance and active, fruits that are bitter astringent and spicy are best. The following list will make a difference in your quest to overcome infertility naturally:

artichoke	garlic	peas
asparagus	horseradish	radishes
beets	kale	rutabaga
broccoli	kohlrabi	spinach
cabbage	leeks	sprouts
carrots	lettuce	squash
cauliflower	mushrooms	tomatoes
celery	okra	turnip
corn	onions	watercress
eggplant	parsley	

Dairy

Replace dairy milk (goat's milk, cow's milk etc) with almond milk. Cow's milk is harder to digest in the human system and it creates a build up of toxins that result in gas and bloating, which is why being vegan makes life simple.

Nuts

Nuts are not advisable since they contain a high content of oil. Stay away from them.

Oils

Stick to freshly pressed almond, sesame and sunflower oil.

Spices and Condiments

Use the following spices:

fenugreek	black pepper	nutmeg
caraway	bay leaf	marjoram
turmeric	mint	orange peel
parsley	paprika	asafetida
ginger	tarragon	cloves
garlic	anise	almond extract
oregano	dill	star anise
basil	cardamom	cumin
rosemary	saffron	coriander
thyme	cinnamon	mustard seeds
curry leaves	peppermint	lots of cayenne

Eat the vegetables that you like and you want to, but whenever you feel down and you feel like you are out of sorts, or if you start gaining weight, switch over to these items and you will see most of the issues disperse.

The HNB Diet

For those of you who fall under the HNB category you will find that you have a rapid constitution. You digest your food quickly and you feel that you are constantly hungry and that you never seem to gain weight.

There are a number of weight gaining supplements that seek to pump you with synthetically derived products. Do not touch them. You have a higher metabolic rate and you have high-energy output. Your body generates the energy whether you like it or not. The best way for you to handle this is to do it with the natural food you eat. One of the favorite things you like is sugar, because you find that sugar gives you the most bang for your nutritional buck. But keep in mind that processed sugar is not a wise choice.

The good thing about having a high metabolic rate is that you are the picture of health. You can almost eat anything and get a way with it, and ice creams are something you can eat all day. By burning almost everything you eat, you even burn toxins that in the food and the rest of your body has gotten used to that. If that metabolic rate increases, or decreases, essentially going out of balance, you will start to catch various issues, including anger, frustration, hot flashes, eczema, and lack of energy.

Eat in small portions and eat frequently. That is the best way to keep you going. The foods that will help you balance your high rate of metabolism are foods that are sweet - which will sustain your rate; foods that are astringent - that will reduce the water, which could reduce your metabolic rate too much; bitter foods to balance the sweetening of your blood.

To feed your metabolic rate, sweet should come from sweet and ripe fruits that are in season, and natural maple syrup. Drink plenty of fresh fruit juices and eat as much watermelons, apples, and mangoes. This is comprehensive list of the fruits that you can have regularly:

apricots	dates	only sweet oranges
berries	sweet grapes and	pears
cherries	raisins	plums
coconuts	melons	prunes

Make sure they fully ripe, in season and sweet. If the fruit is sour it will increase your stomach acidity. Do not favor citrus fruits.

Vegetables

For the same reasons as the fruits favor these vegetables:

artichoke	cabbage	peas
acorn squash	cauliflower	peppers
and zucchini.	celery	potatoes
artichoke	cilantro/coriander	pumpkin
asparagus	cucumber	rutabaga
bell pepper	dandelion greens	scallopini squash
bitter melon	green beans	spaghetti squash
black olives	kale	summer squash
broccoli	leafy greens	sweet
brussel sprouts	lettuce	sweet and white
burdock root	mushrooms	taro root
butternut squash	okra	watercress
	parsley	wheatgrass sprouts
	parsnips	winter squash

Dairy

Stay away from dairy and switch to soy milk and milk from almond and rice milk. Refer to Chapter 6 for ways to make milk.

Legumes

Tofu and tempeh are a great source of protein for HNBs. Along with that here are a few other legumes that you can freely consume:

black beans	lima beans	pinto beans
black-eyed peas	mung beans	soybeans
chickpeas	navy beans	split peas
kidney beans	peas	

Oils

Do not consume and refined oils, especially if you are HNB. The aggravate the metabolic fire to the point of overheating. Freshly pressed sunflower oil, extra virgin olive oil, and walnut oil are best for you. Stay away from ingesting coconut and avocado oil.

Meat

Meats are especially bad for HNBs because of the heat source from the fats. Adopt a vegan lifestyle and stick to it.

Herbal Tea
The following herbal teas will keep you calm during, adequately
hydrated and cool during the day:

alfalfa	fennel	nettle
barley	ginger	oat straw
blackberry	hibiscus	passion
borage	hops	flower
burdock	jasmine	peppermint
catnip	lavender	raspberry
chamomile	lemon balm	red clover
chicory	lemon grass	sarsaparilla
comfrey	liquorice	spearmint
dandelion	marshmallow	strawberry

The SNB Diet

Those within the SNB group are quick, aggressive (in a good way) and
sharp. They are achievers that can push all the other two types to do
well. But to truly take advantage of their inner power, they need
meditation to a higher degree to stabilize their character. This is also
the best way for SNBs to overcome infertility.

From a body frame perspective, SNBs are naturally slimmer. If
imbalanced, they will lose or gain weight and this is a sure sign that
they life is off track. You appreciate chocolates, especially during your
time of the month. You will do well with vegan chocolates, but you are
not adapted for a vegan lifestyle. You need to get your protein from
eggs as tofu and soy bean are not something you can handle well.

Foods that don't suite you will result in gas, bloating, constipation and
irritability and will lead to anxiety and nervousness.

Your forgiving nature is the key to your mental health. Pardon gentles
all as Shakespeare says, and you have mastered that trait to your
benefit. When you are in balances, this always works in your favor.

Stay away from alcohol and caffeine as they are the culprits that totally destabilize you.

When unbalanced you are prone to anxiety and insomnia. Herbal teas help to alleviate that.

Nutrition

You do well with food that is sour, salty and sweet. Use sea salt and unprocessed honey and use fruits for an energy boost. Fruits that are sweet/sour are best. Stay away from astringent fruits, it will make your bowel movement irregular and constipated.

Fruits

These are the fruits that will help to balance you:

grapefruit	oranges	plums
partially ripe mangoes	bananas	avocados
rhubarb	pineapple	kiwifruit
lemons	papaya	berries
sour grapes	apricots	cherries
limes	figs	coconut
melons	peaches	dates
apples	strawberries	

Beverages

Herbal teas that calm and sooth and are best for you. Try these:

liquorice	comfrey	fenugreek
clove	sarsaparilla	marshmallow
catnip	elder flower	chamomile
chicory	penny	lemongrass
hawthorn	sage	ginger
royal	lavender	fennel
straw	eucalyptus	chrysanthemum
orange peel	saffron	peppermint

Oils

Sesame oil and olive oil work best for you but you can also enjoy:

almonds oil	hazelnut oil	pine nut oil
brazil nut oil	peanut oil	pistachio oil
cashew oil	pecan oil	

These are also the ingredients that you can include in making your power bars that are coated in honey. You can also add prunes and raisins.

Vegetables
You can eat all vegetables, but the moment you feel out of balance switch to these and favor them throughout the year:

zucchini	cucumber	asparagus
green chillies	green beans	peas
pumpkin	spaghetti	fennel
rutabaga	potatoes	leeks
radishes	beets	squash
garlic	okra	
watercress	parsnip	

These diets are not meant to move you away from what you have already adopted in the past chapters of this book. These are diets that will hep you get stabilized and balanced in the event something happens in your life that tends to take you off track. Life is not static and we must always count on something happening that removes us from our projected course. We must learn to return our selves back on course. It is like a ship that is sailing on open waters cannot hope to have calms seas and stable winds for its entire journey, the ships captain must neither reject that possibility or let wind and tide determine his course, he has a rudder and his sails to make adjustments and stay the course, as must you. Your rudder and your sail are your meditation and your diet.

With all the overwhelming issues that have surfaced over the course of this book it is perfectly alright that you feel a little overwhelmed. That is alright. But you do know very well up to this point what you have to do. Just breath.

The one thing that would probably have made it clear by now is how far humanity has strayed from nature. This is the single most damming cause of all our ails. The human body has developed itself over the course of millions of years and in that time we have managed to remain happy and content with our existence. However, it is only now where undue stress has taken over our lives because we life in a reality that is not jiving with our nature.

The answer is not to seclude ourselves or turn to asceticism, but rather to embrace everything around us, while strengthening the core of our being. We are not here to change the world and so the problems of the world are not ours to bear. We are hear to change and grow from our own experience. As Gandhi once said, "You must be the change you wish to see in the world." Keeping this in mind at the eve of becoming pregnant, you must understand that that's the world you want to give your child.

One of the psychological barriers that sometimes subconsciously blocks you from conceiving is that you know deep down inside that this world is a tough place for the next generation. From the pollution in the air, to the pollution of our waters and the contamination of our food supply, we have see that the environment is going to get harder for our children. But do not let that scuttle your true purpose on this earth – which is to continue humanity one baby at a time. Your instinct to get pregnant is a strong one, and it is correct.

Chapter 9: The Art of Becoming One

Beating temporary infertility is not about restricting your life. It is about enjoying what life has to offer rather than what commerce and media depicts it to be. You are not loosing out by doing any of the things that have been described so far. You are about to make a huge change in your life, but you should only do so once you realize it to be true in your heart.

You are almost at the end of this book, and you should now learn how to connect with your spouse. So far you have gotten to know him, by his presence. When he massaged you and you massaged him, you focused on getting to know his presence.

You then got to know him when you practiced your combined meditation. That is a deeply moving experience and you will begin to understand all the things that motivate him – from his joys to his fears. When you get to know him, you will also get to understand him, and when you do, forgiving him for his sins becomes easier. After all we are prone to mistakes as well, don't we wish someone would understand that too? Well that is his job, to understand you and forgive you, and it is your job to understand him and forgive him – no matter how serious you think the transgression is.

Form there you have reached the point that you have gotten to know him and he has known you approximately two thirds of the way. But still that is a significantly more than what most people ever know. Now it is time for you to complete the remaining one third and close the gap that remains between the two of you. This is the final task in overcoming fertility.

A Combined Effort

To overcome infertility it is a combined effort. The two of you must bridge this gap together and by the time you get here, if you had followed all the necessary steps, you will find this last step pleasurable and extremely gratifying. It is an energy that fosters the conception beyond anything you have ever realized.

This is more than just sex. This is the art of two bodies combining to become one in action and sealing the oneness in spirit. It is the consummation of the two to become one. Please make sure your spouse reads this so that both of you can attain what is truly needed.

Preparing the Union

When the union is contemplated for the first time you need to be in a position of purity and anticipation. There should be at least one month of celibacy by both of you and it should be a commitment that is not broken by either of you, even in private.

In this month, you diets should be unbroken, your meditation, both individual and combined, should be smoothly regular, your water fasts should be regular and you should be in balance with the aid of the foods that have been designed for each body type. You should also be working out everyday. You are, at this point glowing and the picture of health. You are more aware of what is gong in you and around you more than any other time in your life.
With this ready, you are about to take the first step. You do not need to calculate your ovulation cycle. If you are keeping mindful of your body, you will automatically know when you are ovulating and what your body is doing. If you are following the advice or smelling natural, your spouse will instinctively know when you are ovulating, because his senses are designed to pick up on it. So there is no need to calculate. Leave it to your body and his senses to figure it out. The key here is to not use any artificial perfumes that will confuse and mask the senses and the scents.

Taking the First Step

The first step and the few more after this are dry runs. It is a process of waking up something deep down inside both of you. You will see the union catch fire with this process and you will grow to love each other deeper than any feeling of infatuation that may have existed on that first date.

Begin with the same massage that you have done in Chapter 4. By this point, your spouse knows where all your pressure points are and he knows exactly how much pressure to use. You are the same.

Begin with the feet and move on to the calves applying just the right pressure that will help to release the endorphins and empty the lymph nodes in the this the shoulders and the pelvic area. Spend more time in the inner thighs and more time in the hips. Massage the lower belly and move up to the stomach. In the earlier massage more prominence was given to the back. In this exercise more focus is given to the front.

There are seven areas that wake up a women's senses and prepares her for unification with her spouse.

The Physical Touch

The physical touch helps to release the endorphins and begin the journey. It is the beginning of the physical communication. Use the palms and the a firm grip to communicate.

Skin

The first and most important part of a women is her skin. Whether it is the skin in her scalp, or the skin at the base of her feet, our skin is an important part of letting someone in to our lives. If the person means nothing to us, nothing they do will wake up the skin. But when a person means more to us than we realize, the skin shows it. The touch on the skin now is one that is light and breezy. Your partner must massage you with the gentleness of the tips of his fingers so that his energy will permeate your skin. The tips of the fingers are a formidable ally in this area.

The Ears

The ears are to be tenderly touched and massaged. There is no kissing or introduction of anything except his fingers.

The Face

The face has a number of points that are receptive to your spouses gentle touch. Among these include the lips, the cheeks, the forehead, and the temples.

The Neck
The neck is the shortest way to the brain and it is also full of sensitive nerve endings that deserve to awaken. First use palms for a firm massage, then switch to finger tips for a gentle stroke. The touch must be so light that there is almost no contact being made.

The Breasts
The breasts are usually very tender and gentle if it is the second last thing to be approached. Remember the best way to awaken a woman's body is to do it in steps. Do not jump from the skin to the breasts in one leap, it will reduce the effectiveness. No matter how sensitive and ready you think you are, make sure your spouse follows this path.

The Mound
The final area is the mound and the surrounding area. There are numerous nerve endings here and it is the area that is fired up by the stimulation of everything else. By the time this area is touched, it should be well stimulated by the touch of the other areas.

Firm Grip
These seven areas are to be approached in the following sequence: begin with the deep tissue massage, followed by the touch of the skin in all areas of the body from the fingers to the palms to the writs to the fore arms and even the armpits and the crease of the knee. Make sure that the shoulders are gripped firmly and the inner thighs are held as well.

Light Touch
Once the entire body has been massaged firmly, it is time to allow the light touch of the skin to commence. The light touch creates an imperceptible bond that ignites the deepest connection between two people. The touch is something that, when you combine it with the meditation, creates an almost instant attachment of body and soul. The light touch is more powerful than a bear hug. The light touch awakens

and increases the sensitivity.

There is no detailed course of action here because you will play it as it happens and this is one area that should not be scripted. The point is that you start with a firm grip then you move to the light touch. The light touch should be spread across the body and especially across the neck, descending to the breasts then the pelvic area.

The first time this is done, stop after the light touch and remain in an embrace for the duration of the remaining night until morning. You can do this every night and relish in the fact that the orgasm is not the point of true intercourse. The orgasm actually robs you from the moment if it is not allowed to reach its crescendo in due course.

Continue this practice until you feel more parts of your body awaken. The idea is to awaken the spirit of the union. It also teaches the man, that contrary to what civilization has touted all this while, there is more to a women then just the opportunity for an orgasm.

Multiple repetitions of this will increase the height of sensitivity and shows you the different areas of the physical and spiritual body that you have not seen before.

Point to Note: Do not use this technique for entertainment. This is the physical manifestation of true love between a man and a women who are about to create a new life. It is deeply sensual and if the two people are not in a committed relationship, the break-up will be catastrophic for one or both parties.

If you do not have the benefit of meditation and the increased powers of your mind, it would be impossible to contain the level of sensual attraction between the two of you. Do not succumb yet. Once the time has elapsed, what you will find and what you should expect is that the bond between the two of you has increased. You will realize that the myopic and pubescent thought of reaching an orgasm was not only puerile but also selfish. It also missed the plot. There is something a lot more to this relationship then the sudden explosion of pleasure.

In your quest to overcome infertility you will realize that the best way to do it is to fall deeply in unison with your partner and this unification is not just sexual. It is physical, it is psychological and it is the process of becoming one. Reaching an orgasm is the antithesis of this. But do not despair if you are still wanting to achieve the climax. Years of programming from the world is not going to change you overnight. But if you reflect and look deep within your own heart, you will know this to be true. The idea of chasing after an orgasm after 5 minutes of rough handling will begin to repulse you.

Chapter 10 The Art of Staying as One

The art of becoming one takes three steps. You are now at step two. The process of unification is the last in a series of overcoming infertility and as you can already tell it is a two person endeavour. If you thought you were in it yourself, then you just had the awakening of a lifetime.

Point to Note: If your spouse has been sceptical about following you on this journey, that is fine, but if your spouse has been blocking you off at every juncture, like not wanting to get closer to you or not understanding the need to participate in the meditation exercises. You have a way out of this. You need to be true to yourself and if he indeed is not ready for a child, it is time for you to understand and forgive him for it.

Unfortunately, there will be some of you who find out that there are some relationships that are not meant to be. If that is the case, then that is the main reason you are not able to naturally conceive. Do not be afraid to make a decision at this point. Find out of your spouse is truly uncomfortable or they just don't want to have a child. It is still possible to adopt and if that is what is meant to be, then that would be a good way to go.

However, if your spouse has come all this way with you and the two of you have bridged most of the gap then you have a very good chance of getting pregnant and raising a well balanced and healthy child. Do not be surprised if this process takes up to two years to materialize and get to this point.

The art of staying as one is not as complex or complicated as it is made out to be. You must understand that the reason a man and a women don't initially understand each other is because we are totally different. But that difference is not to make us suspect each other. The two of you need to be different to complement each other not be the same and make the same mistakes together. We all have our weaknesses. I have mine and my spouse has his, without me he would make all the same mistakes, and without him I would make all the same ones I've made in the past. Together, we have transcended the puerile world and became parents to well adjusted children. But we couldn't do that without learning how to stay as one.

Back to the Art

After a few weeks of firm grip and light touch exercises, you will start to appreciate the awakening. It is not totally describable in words and it is truly personal and individual, but one thing you will appreciate is the increased bond between the two of you.

The next part of the exercise now moves to the next phase. In this phase there will be no focus on orgasms as well. Remember, in a true relationship the idea and pleasure comes from true unification, and the way to overcome infertility is to look past the simplicity of an orgasm.

In this stage the idea is to begin as you have always done prior to this but this time it is for you to move more attention to the breasts and the pelvic area. The woman's pelvic area is the cradle of humanity. It deserves to be treated that way and not disrespected. Massage it constantly and remain in the moment, do not yearn for the orgasm and forsake the moment in its pursuit. You should be aware of every breath he makes and totally keep him in your sphere. If you can feel the fire in your chest from the breathing, envelope him with this flame.

The detail of how he should touch you are not the point of this book, but it is sufficient to remind you that there should be no orgasm.

When you focus on the pelvic are, the idea of deep stimulation is to get the pelvic area and the contents inside including the ovaries and the uterus to get ready to receive your partner. This means a number of things. It is not just the softening of the tissue and the opening of the cavities, but on a deeper level, it is about creating a hospitable environment for his share of the union. If your uterus is inhospitable there will be no way any of his DNA carriers are going to be able to penetrate your defences.

By stimulating the pelvic area you are creating a bond deep within you. At this point you should begin to connect at the lips. The hands should be used for embrace at this point and there is no longer the need to apply firm pressure or gentle touches. The point to make physical connection has arrived and you should be engaged in kissing. This is the step that is the step before the final consummation.

Kissing is an important part of the union and should not be taken lightly. Many women who are in tune with themselves are usually taken, or swept off their feet, by the kiss that can seem to tell them a lot. It can, but it should be at this point that the kiss is used to initiate the final step.

The kiss opens the woman to the possibility of being fertile. The kiss, if strong enough can create the necessary conditions for ovulation even if the calendar is not in the proper time. The kiss can and should go on for hours. But not forced just because the book says it. It should be something where the two of you loose your individual self in the union. It shows your mind and spirit the location of the union. The kiss must be like nothing else shared by any other person and you or any other person and the father of your child. This is no ordinary kiss.

This session, the first step in the last of the unification will go on for a few days. When you meet anybody the next day, they will see a noticeable difference in your appearance. They will see a glow that was never present and you will feel that glow too.

You are finally at the stage of final bonding. You begin with the massage and get to he point of the kissing and you prepare for the point of unification. Your vaginal track is ready to receive and it has softened. The introduction should be made, but once again there should be no attempt made at an orgasm. By this point you already see the benefits of this.

Chose the position that is most comfortable for you and both of you can begin by being mindful of your breathing. Allow the penetration to be done slowly but do no do the usually gyration. It should be a gentler entry and a unification. There is no need to thrust and release. Your spouse should enter you, or you should envelope him and stop. That unification should be combined with the kissing and the embrace. The union should be graceful.

Continue to do this for a few more days – not necessarily everyday. But continue these sessions a few more times until you find yourself completely comfortable with the physical union. Then when you are both ready, do your breathing and enter the state of combined meditation while you are physically united.

This will complete the journey. Those bonds the couple and makes it one. This completes your quest for overcoming infertility. What remains is the release of his DNA to join yours.
On the day you ovulate, you will feel it and he will know it. When you follow all the steps to the point of introduction, and stay in that state, and in the state of combined meditation, you will both achieve a sensation that is so much greater than any orgasm you have previously felt. It is so much more that it is not appropriate to even call it by that name. The orgasm and release will be triggered by the ovulation and the chemistry of your uterus which will lead your spouse to release his contribution. You will both know the moment and you will feel it while you are in the state of combined meditation. From here forth, this will be your preferred way to unite and you will see this change the way you live.

Most people mistake sex as entertainment and as a way to feel loved and feel the moment of affection. If you've noticed the end of sex, especially the ones that last all of ten minutes leaves you drained and not totally confident of yourself. It happens in both, men and women, but it is more acute with us because we are more sensitive to it. But if you ask a man, the macho ego of self will preclude his true admission to surface.

Conclusion

This book has thought you that to overcome infertility it requires that you undertake a holistic makeover that includes revitalizing your physical body and rejuvenating your psychology and converting some of the definitions you have come to hold as the truth. You have realized that infertility is not just a woman's issue, or a man's. It is the two individual's union that is shared. An otherwise healthy man and a healthy woman who are not in physical, mental and emotional union would not always be able to conceive.

The idea of becoming pregnant is not limited to the conscious decision two people make. The thousands of unplanned' pregnancies that do occur after all the precaution and prevention they have taken is one proof of this. So are the millions of people who are trying so hard to become parents they forgot to become bonded first. Pregnancy is more than just what we learned in biology class. It is more than just a physical process. It is, for lack of a better word, a spiritual process. (Note: spiritual does not mean religious)

Your Free Gift

I wanted to show my appreciation for your purchase so I have put together a free gift for you!

Easy to follow Get Pregnant Faster Exercise Summary

Just visit

http://newwheelpublishing.com/getpregnantfaster

to download it now

I know you'll love this Gift.

Thanks!

Cecilia Suares

Enjoyed this book?

Thank you so much for your support!

If you enjoyed this book, I'd be grateful if you'd post a short review. Your support really does make a difference and I read all the reviews personally so I can get your feedback and make this book even better.

I would love to hear from you because I really value your support, feedback and insight so I can better serve you in the near future.

Thank you so much!

-Cecilia Suares